How to Boost Your Immune System
Healthy Ways to Strengthen Your Immune System

Copyright © 2020

DEDICATION

Contents

Immune System Explained

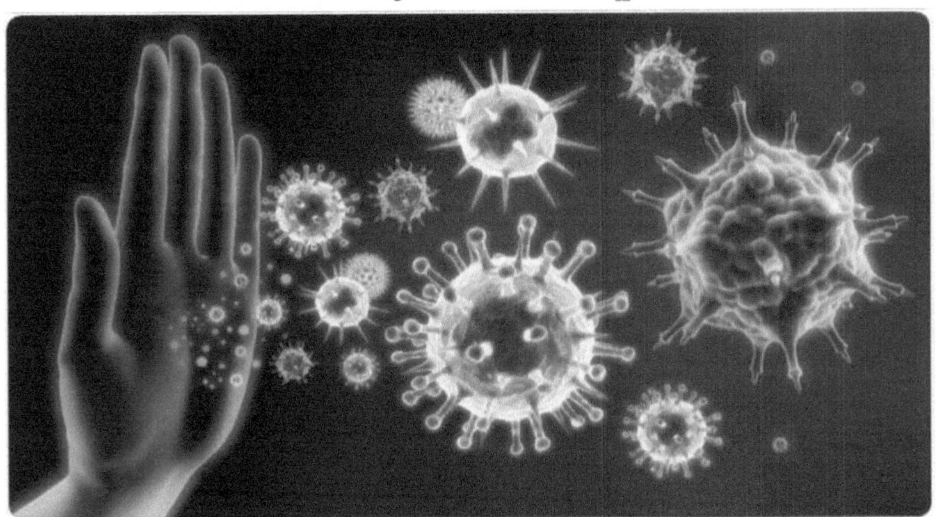

The immune system is made up of special organs, cells and chemicals that fight infection (microbes). The main parts of the immune system are: white blood cells, antibodies, the complement system, the lymphatic system, the spleen, the thymus, and the bone marrow. These are the parts of your immune system that actively fight infection.

The immune system and microbial infection

The immune system keeps a record of every microbe it has ever defeated, in types of white blood cells (B- and T-lymphocytes) known as memory cells. This means it can recognise and destroy the microbe quickly if it enters the body again, before it can multiply and make you feel sick.

Some infections, like the flu and the common cold, have to be fought many times because so many different viruses or strains of the same type of virus can cause these illnesses. Catching a cold or flu from one virus does not give you immunity against the others.

Parts of the immune system

The main parts of the immune system are:

- white blood cells
- antibodies
- complement system
- lymphatic system
- spleen
- bone marrow
- thymus.

White blood cells

White blood cells are the key players in your immune system. They are made in your bone marrow and are part of the lymphatic system.

White blood cells move through blood and tissue throughout your body, looking for foreign invaders (microbes) such as bacteria, viruses, parasites and fungi. When they find them, they launch an immune attack.

White blood cells include lymphocytes (such as B-cells, T-cells and natural killer cells), and many other types of immune cells.

Antibodies

Antibodies help the body to fight microbes or the toxins (poisons) they produce. They do this by recognising substances called antigens on the surface of the microbe, or in the chemicals they produce, which mark the microbe or toxin as being foreign. The antibodies then mark these antigens for destruction. There are many cells, proteins and chemicals involved in this attack.

Complement system

The complement system is made up of proteins whose actions complement the work done by antibodies.

Lymphatic system

The lymphatic system is a network of delicate tubes throughout the body. The main roles of the lymphatic system are to:

- manage the fluid levels in the body
- react to bacteria
- deal with cancer cells
- deal with cell products that otherwise would result in disease or disorders
- absorb some of the fats in our diet from the intestine.

The lymphatic system is made up of:

- lymph nodes (also called lymph glands) -- which trap microbes
- lymph vessels -- tubes that carry lymph, the colourless fluid that bathes your body's tissues and contains infection-fighting white blood cells
- white blood cells (lymphocytes).

Spleen

The spleen is a blood-filtering organ that removes microbes and destroys old or damaged red blood cells. It also makes disease-fighting components of the immune system (including antibodies and lymphocytes).

Bone marrow

Bone marrow is the spongy tissue found inside your bones. It produces the red blood cells our bodies need to carry oxygen, the white blood cells we use to fight infection, and the platelets we need to help our blood clot.

Thymus

The thymus filters and monitors your blood content. It produces the white blood cells called T-lymphocytes.

The body's other defences against microbes

As well as the immune system, the body has several other ways to defend itself against microbes, including:

- skin - a waterproof barrier that secretes oil with bacteria-killing properties
- lungs - mucous in the lungs (phlegm) traps foreign particles, and small hairs (cilia) wave the mucous upwards so it can be coughed out
- digestive tract - the mucous lining contains antibodies, and the acid in the stomach can kill most microbes
- other defences - body fluids like skin oil, saliva and tears contain anti-bacterial enzymes that help reduce the risk of infection. The constant flushing of the urinary tract and the

bowel also helps.

Fever is an immune system response

A rise in body temperature, or fever, can happen with some infections. This is actually an immune system response. A rise in temperature can kill some microbes. Fever also triggers the body's repair process.

Common disorders of the immune system

It is common for people to have an over- or underactive immune system.

Overactivity of the immune system can take many forms, including:

- allergic diseases - where the immune system makes an overly strong response to allergens. Allergic diseases are very common. They include allergies to foods, medications or stinging insects, anaphylaxis (life-threatening allergy), hay fever (allergic rhinitis), sinus disease, asthma, hives (urticaria), dermatitis and eczema

- autoimmune diseases - where the immune system mounts a response against normal components of the body. Autoimmune diseases range from common to rare. They include multiple sclerosis, autoimmune thyroid disease, type 1 diabetes, systemic lupus erythematosus, rheumatoid arthritis and systemic vasculitis.

Underactivity of the immune system, also called immunodeficiency, can:

- be inherited - examples of these conditions include primary immunodeficiency diseases such as common variable immunodeficiency (CVID), x-linked severe combined immunodeficiency (SCID) and complement deficiencies
- arise as a result of medical treatment - this can occur due to medications such as corticosteroids or chemotherapy
- be caused by another disease - such as HIV/AIDS or certain types of cancer.

An underactive immune system does not function correctly and makes people vulnerable to infections. It can be life threatening in severe cases.

People who have had an organ transplant need immunosuppression treatment to prevent the body from attacking the transplanted organ.

Immunoglobulin therapy

Immunoglobulins (commonly known as antibodies) are used to treat people who are unable to make enough of their own, or whose antibodies do not work properly. This treatment is known as immunoglobulin therapy.

Until recently, immunoglobulin therapy in Australia mostly involved delivery of immunoglobulins through a drip into the vein – known as intravenous immunoglobulin (IVIg) therapy. Now, subcutaneous immunoglobulin (SCIg) can be delivered into the fatty tissue under the skin, which may offer benefits for some patients. This is known as subcutaneous infusion or SCIg therapy.

Subcutaneous immunoglobulin is similar to intravenous

immunoglobulin. It is made from plasma – the liquid part of blood containing important proteins like antibodies.

Many health services are now offering SCIg therapy to eligible patients with specific immune conditions. If you are interested, please discuss your particular requirements with your treating specialist.

Immunisation

Immunisation works by copying the body's natural immune response. A vaccine (a small amount of a specially treated virus, bacterium or toxin) is injected into the body. The body then makes antibodies to it.

If a vaccinated person is exposed to the actual virus, bacterium or toxin, they won't get sick because their body will recognise it and know how to attack it successfully. Vaccinations are available against many diseases, including measles and tetanus.

The immunisations you may need are decided by your health, age, lifestyle and occupation. Together, these factors are referred to as HALO, which is defined as:

- health - some health conditions or factors may make you more vulnerable to vaccine-preventable diseases. For example, premature birth, asthma, diabetes, heart, lung, spleen or kidney conditions, Down syndrome and HIV will mean you may benefit from additional or more frequent immunisations
- age - at different ages you need protection from different vaccine-preventable diseases. Australia's National Immunisation Program sets out recommended immunisations for babies, children, older people and other people at risk, such as

Aboriginal and Torres Strait Islanders. Most recommended vaccines are available at no cost to these groups

- lifestyle - lifestyle choices can have an impact on your immunisation needs. Travelling overseas to certain places, planning a family, sexual activity, smoking, and playing contact sport that may expose you directly to someone else's blood, will mean you may benefit from additional or more frequent immunisations

- occupation - you are likely to need extra immunisations, or need to have them more often, if you work in an occupation that exposes you to vaccine-preventable diseases or puts you into contact with people who are more susceptible to problems from vaccine-preventable diseases (such as babies or young children, pregnant women, the elderly, and people with chronic or acute health conditions). For example, if you work in aged care, childcare, healthcare, emergency services or sewerage repair and maintenance, discuss your immunisation needs with your doctor. Some employers help with the cost of relevant vaccinations for their employees.

The Immune System and Cancer

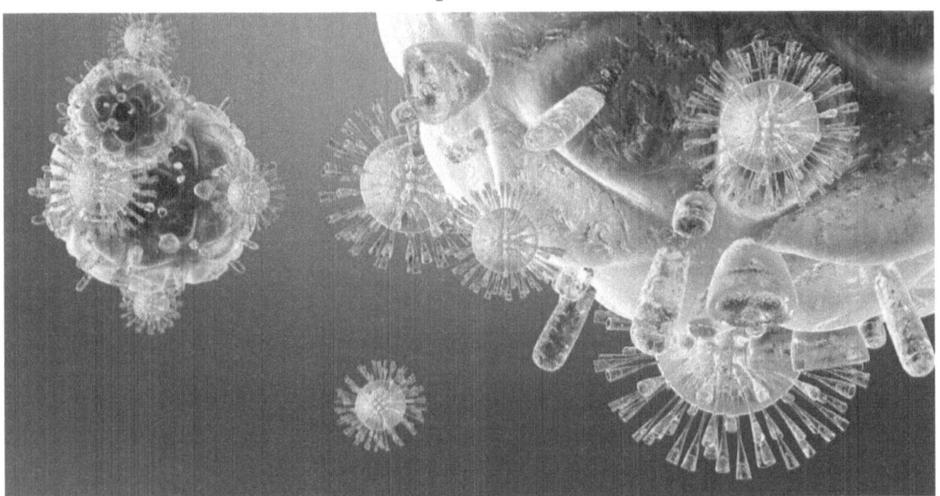

What the immune system does

The immune system protects the body against illness and infection that bacteria, viruses, fungi or parasites can cause. It is a collection of reactions and responses that the body makes to damaged cells or infection. So it is sometimes called the immune response.

The immune system is important to people with cancer because:

cancer can weaken the immune system

cancer treatments might weaken the immune system

the immune system may help to fight cancer

Cancer and treatments may weaken immunity

Cancer can weaken the immune system by spreading into the bone marrow. Open a glossary item The bone marrow makes blood cells that help to fight infection. This happens most often in leukaemia or lymphoma, but it can happen with other cancers too. The cancer can stop the bone marrow from making so many blood cells.

Certain cancer treatments can temporarily weaken the immune system. This is because they can cause a drop in the number of white blood cells made in the bone marrow. Cancer treatments that are more likely to weaken the immune system are:

chemotherapy

targeted cancer drugs

radiotherapy

high dose of steroids

The immune system can help to fight cancer

Some cells of the immune system can recognise cancer cells as abnormal and kill them. But this may not be enough to get rid of a cancer altogether.

Some treatments aim to use the immune system to fight cancer.

There are 2 main parts of the immune system:

the protection we have from birth (in built immune protection)

the protection we develop after having certain diseases (acquired immunity)

In built immune protection

This is also called innate immunity. These mechanisms are always ready and prepared to defend the body from infection. They can act immediately (or very quickly). This in built protection comes from:

a barrier formed by the skin around the body

the inner linings of the gut and lungs, which produce mucus and trap invading bacteria

hairs that move the mucus and trapped bacteria out of the lungs

stomach acid, which kills bacteria

helpful bacteria growing in the bowel, which prevent other bacteria from taking over

urine flow, which flushes bacteria out of the bladder and urethra

white blood cells called neutrophils, which can find and kill bacteria

Different things can overcome and damage these natural protection mechanisms. For example:

something may break the skin barrier, such as having a drip in your arm or a wound from surgery

a catheter into your bladder can become a route for bacteria to get inside the bladder and cause infection

anti acid medicines for heartburn may neutralise the stomach acid that kills bacteria

Certain cancer treatments can also overcome these protection mechanisms. Chemotherapy can temporarily reduce the number of neutrophils in the body, making it harder for you to fight infections. Radiotherapy to the lung can damage the hairs and mucus producing cells that help to remove bacteria.

Neutrophils

Neutrophils are a type of white blood cell that are very important for fighting infection. They can:

move to areas of infection in the body

stick to the invading bacteria, viruses or fungi

swallow up the bacteria, viruses or fungi and kill them with chemicals

When you don't have enough neutrophils in your blood, doctors may say that you are neutropaenic.

Chemotherapy, targeted cancer drugs and some radiotherapy treatments can lower the number of neutrophils in the blood. So you might get more bacterial or fungal infections after these treatments.

It is important for you to know the following when having cancer treatment:

infections can become serious very quickly in people with low neutrophil counts

antibiotics could save your life so if you get a fever or feel ill phone your advice line or go to hospital straight away

you might need to take antibiotics to help prevent severe infection if your blood counts are low

It is more usual to become ill from bugs you carry around with you than from catching someone else's. This means that you shouldn't have to avoid contact with your family, friends or children after treatment.

You can ask your doctor or nurse what precautions you should take against infection.

Acquired immunity

This is immune protection that the body learns after having certain diseases. The body learns to recognise each different kind of bacteria, fungus or virus it meets for the first time. So the next time the same bug invades the body it is easier for the immune system to fight it. This is why you usually only get some infectious diseases such as measles or chicken pox once.

Vaccination works by using this type of immunity. A vaccine contains a small amount of protein from a disease. This is not harmful but it allows the immune system to recognise the disease if it meets it again. The immune response can then stop you getting the disease.

Some vaccines use small amounts of the live bacteria or virus. These are live attenuated vaccines. It means that scientists have changed the virus or bacteria so that it stimulates the immune system to make antibodies. A live vaccine won't cause an infection.

Other types of vaccine use killed bacteria or viruses, or parts of proteins that bacteria and viruses produce.

B cells and T cells

Lymphocytes are a type of white blood cells involved in the acquired immune response. There are 2 main types of lymphocytes:

B cells

T cells

The bone marrow produces all blood cells, including B and T lymphocytes. Like the other blood cells, they have to fully mature before they can help in the immune response.

B cells mature in the bone marrow. But T cells mature in the thymus gland. Open a glossary item Once they are mature, the B and T cells travel to the spleen Open a glossary item and lymph nodes Open a glossary item ready to fight infection.

What B cells do

B cells react against invading bacteria or viruses by making proteins called antibodies. Your body makes a different antibody for each different type of germ (bug). The antibody locks onto the surface of the invading bacteria or virus. This marks the invader so that the body knows it is dangerous and needs to be killed. Antibodies can also find and kill damaged cells.

The B cells are part of the memory of the immune system. The next time the same germ tries to invade the B cells that make the right antibody are ready for it. They are able to make their antibody very quickly.

How antibodies work

Antibodies have 2 ends. One end sticks to proteins on the outside of white blood cells. The other end sticks to the germ or damaged cell and helps to kill it. The end of the antibody that sticks to the white blood cell is always the same. Scientists call this the constant end.

The end of the antibody that recognises germs and damaged cells varies, depending on the cell it needs to recognise. So it is called the variable end. Each B cell makes antibodies with a different variable end from other B cells.

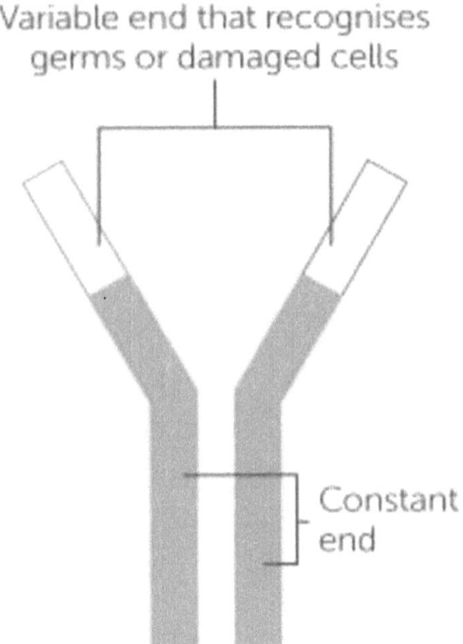

Cancer cells are not normal cells. So some antibodies with variable ends recognise cancer cells and stick to them.

What T cells do

There are different kinds of T cells called:

helper T cells

killer T cells

The helper T cells stimulate the B cells to make antibodies and help killer cells develop.

Killer T cells kill the body's own cells that have been invaded by the viruses or bacteria. This prevents the germ from reproducing in the cell and then infecting other cells.

Cancer treatments that use the immune system

Some cancer treatments use parts of the immune system to help treat cancer.

Immunotherapy

Immunotherapy is a treatment for some types of cancer. It uses the immune system to find and kill cancer cells.

They are helpful in cancer treatment because cancer cells are different from normal cells. And the immune system can recognise and kill abnormal cells.

In the laboratory scientists can produce different chemicals that are part of the immune response. So, they can make different types of immunotherapies such as:

monoclonal antibodies (MABs), which recognise and attack certain proteins on the surface of cancer cells

vaccines to help the immune system to recognise and attack cancer

cytokines to help to boost the immune system

adoptive cell transfer to change the genes in a person's white blood cells

COVID-19 Infection Linked to Overactive Immune Cells

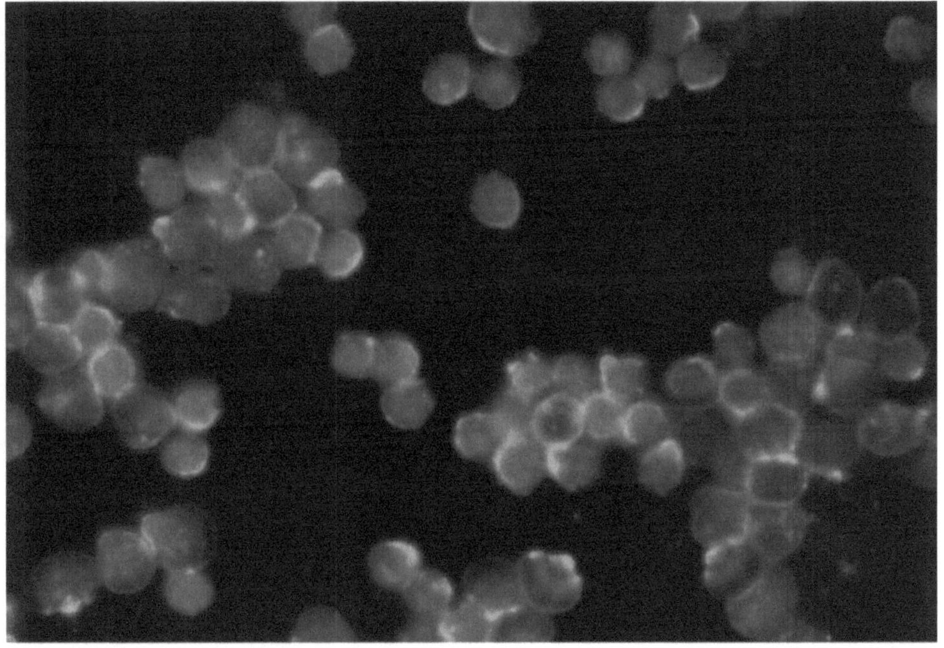

When infected with the SARS-CoV-2 coronavirus, many people experience mild and moderate symptoms, but for some people infection can be severe or fatal. Scientists are urgently seeking to understand how COVID-19 can become severe.

Now, a study led by Imperial College London researchers has revealed how an overreaction of part of the immune system could be linked to severe cases of COVID-19.

When we are infected with pathogens like bacteria and viruses, our bodies mount several types of immune system response. One of the major components are T cells, which come in several different forms that coordinate the immune response, from killing infected cells to recruiting more T cells to the fight.

Sometimes, our immune system overreacts to invaders, for example during an allergic reaction, resulting in T cells killing normal, healthy cells and causing tissue damage. However, there is a 'brake mechanism' that should kick in, causing T cells to reduce their activity and calming inflammation.

Fine detail on the immune system

Researchers tested samples from the lungs of six COVID-19 patients in China with severe symptoms and compared them to samples from three moderate COVID-19 patients and three healthy individuals.

Although the samples were from relatively few patients, the team investigated gene usage in single cells, gaining fine detail on the immune system response. This method allowed them to analyse rare cells and their dynamics, which cannot be achieved with conventional methods.

Failing brakes

The found that the lungs of severe COVID-19 patients had accumulated a broad range of 'hyperactivated' T cells, suggesting the brake mechanism had failed. This overreaction 'paralyses' the overall T cell system, causing it to fail at fighting the virus, as well as causing more damage to the lungs through severe inflammation and tissue destruction.

On closer inspection of the mechanism, the researchers found that the protein 'Foxp3', which usually induced the brake mechanism, is inhibited in lungs of severe COVID-19 patients. They are unsure why Foxp3 is inhibited, but further study could reveal this, and potentially lead to a way to put the brakes back on the T cell response, reducing the severity of the disease.

The Importance of Immunity in Today's World

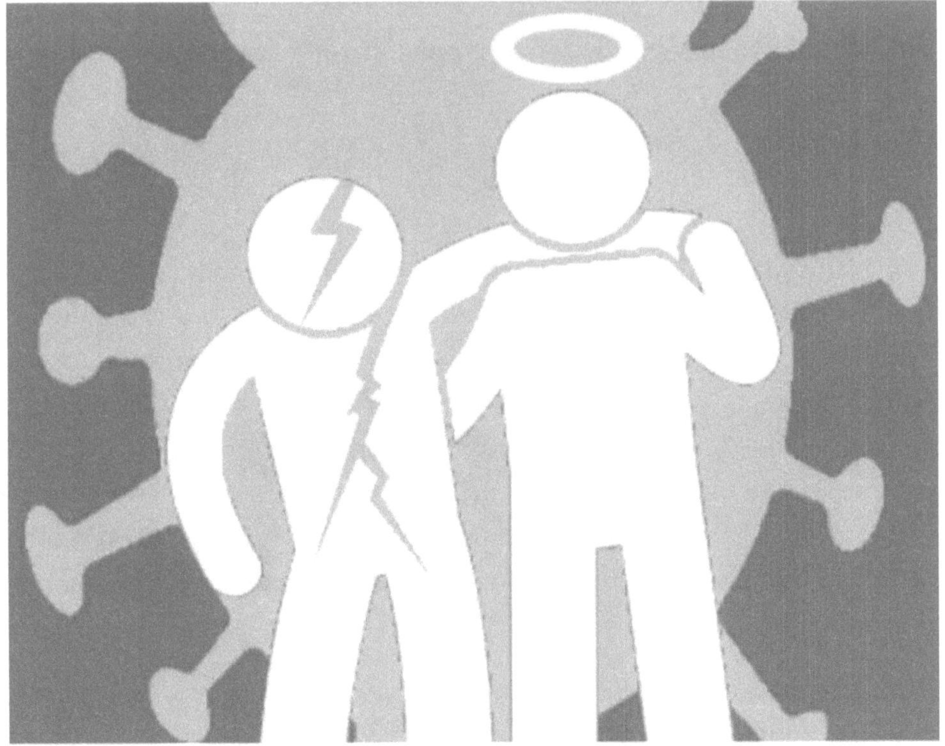

While the global population is growing rapidly, and people are living longer, our living environment has changed substantially. There is therefore a greater need to support our health and wellbeing, primarily our immune system, at different stages throughout our life.

These concerns regarding immunity have become more important, given the periodic outbreaks of infectious diseases such as SARS (Severe acute respiratory syndrome), MERS (Middle East respiratory syndrome), and now the coronavirus pandemic, that within a few months, has led to more than three million cases across the world.

Your immune system works 24/7, whether it's offering you protection from the Coronavirus, a common cold or even pink eye. On the whole, it does a pretty good job, but sometimes it fails: a germ invades successfully and makes you sick.

So what makes up our immune system and what is best way of keeping yours healthy?

Your immune system is an intricate network of cells, tissues, and organs that band together to defend your body against foreign invaders – things like germs, viruses and bacteria. A healthy immune system protects you by creating a barrier that stops those invaders from entering your body. If one happens to slip by, it starts to produce white blood cells and other chemicals that attack and destroy these foreign substances. If your immune system can't get rid of the invader before it starts to reproduce, it simply revs up even more to destroy the invaders as they multiply.

In addition to blood cells and chemicals that physically attack germs, your skin, lungs, digestive tract, saliva and tears are also all involved in the immune response. That's why washing you hands and not touching your face are so important too.

5 Ways to Boost Your Immune System

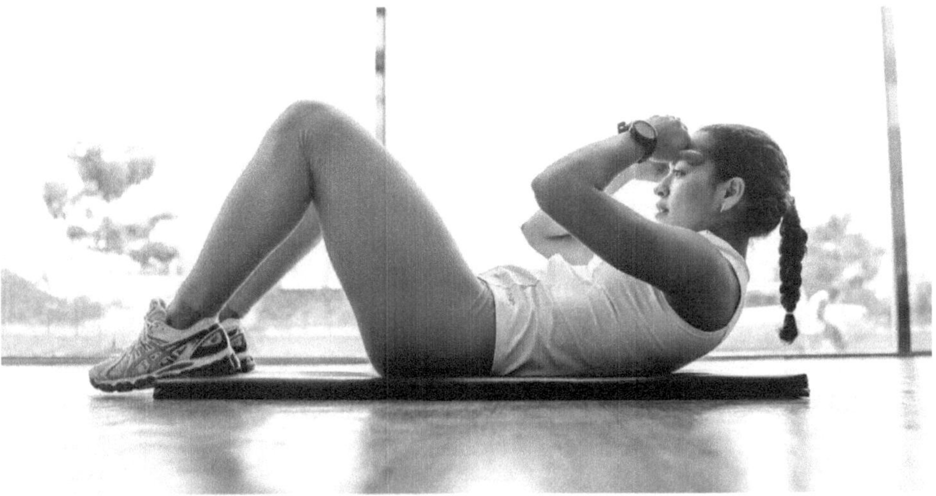

There are plenty of supplements and products in the grocery store that claim to help boost your immune system. But while it may sound like a no-brainer, boosting your immune system is actually much harder to accomplish than you might think — and for good reason.

Your immune system is incredibly complex. It has to be strong enough and sophisticated enough to fight off a variety of illnesses and infections, but not so strong that it overreacts unnecessarily — causing allergies and other autoimmune disorders to develop. To operate in such a delicate balance, your immune system is tightly controlled by a variety of inputs.

But despite its complexity, there are everyday lifestyle habits you can focus on to help give your immune system what it needs to fight off an infection or illness. Here are five science-backed ways to ensure your immune system has everything it needs to function optimally, as well as why you shouldn't rely on supplements to boost your immune system.

Maintain a healthy diet

As with most things in your body, a healthy diet is key to a strong immune system. This means making sure you eat plenty of vegetables, fruits, legumes, whole grains, lean protein and healthy fats.

In addition to providing your immune system the energy it needs, a healthy diet can help ensure you're getting sufficient amounts of the micronutrients that play a role in maintaining your immune system, including:

Vitamin B6, found in chicken, salmon, tuna, bananas, green vegetables and potatoes (with the skin)

Vitamin C, found in citrus fruit, including oranges and strawberries, as well as tomatoes, broccoli and spinach

Vitamin E, found in almonds, sunflower and safflower oil, sunflower seeds, peanut butter and spinach

Since experts believe that your body absorbs vitamins more efficiently from dietary sources, rather than supplements, the best way to support your immune system is to eat a well-balanced diet.

Exercise regularly

Physical activity isn't just for building muscles and helping yourself de-stress — it's also an important part of being healthy and supporting a healthy immune system.

One way exercise may improve immune function is by boosting your overall circulation, making it easier for immune cells and other infection-fighting molecules to travel more easily throughout your body.

In fact, studies have shown that engaging in as little as 30 minutes of moderate-to-vigorous exercise every day helps stimulate your immune system. This means it's important to focus on staying active and getting regular exercise.

Hydrate, hydrate, hydrate

Water plays many important roles in your body, including supporting your immune system. A fluid in your circulatory system called lymph, which carries important infection-fighting immune cells around your body, is largely made up of water. Being dehydrated slows down the movement of lymph, sometimes leading to an impaired immune system.

Even if you're not exercising or sweating, you're constantly losing water through your breath, as well as through your urine and bowel movements. To help support your immune system, be sure you're replacing the water you lose with water you can use — which starts with knowing how much water you really need.

Get plenty of sleep

Sleep certainly doesn't feel like an active process, but there are plenty of important activities happening in your body when you're not awake — even if you don't realize it. For instance, important infection-fighting molecules are created while you sleep.

Studies have shown that people who don't get enough quality sleep are more prone to getting sick after exposure to viruses, such as those that cause the common cold. To give your immune system the best chance to fight off infection and illness, it's important to know how much sleep you should be getting every night, as well as the steps to take if your sleep is suffering.

Minimize stress

Whether it comes on quick or builds over time, it's important to understand how stress affects your health — including the impact it has on your immune system. During a period of stress, particularly chronic stress that's frequent and long-lasting, your body responds by initiating a stress response. This stress response, in turn, suppresses your immune system — increasing your chance of infection or illness.

Stress is different for everyone, and how we relieve it is, too. Given the effect it can have on your health, it's important to know how to identify stress. And, whether it's deep breathing, mediation, prayer or exercise, you should also get familiar with the activities that help you reduce stress.

One last word on supplements

There's no shortage of supplements claiming they can stimulate your immune system — but be wary of these promises.

First thing's first, there's no evidence that supplements actually help improve your immune system or your chances of fighting off an infection or illness. In addition, unlike medications, supplements aren't regulated or approved by the FDA. For instance, if you think a megadose of vitamin C can help you keep from getting sick, think again.

If you're looking for ways to help boost your immune system, consider keeping up with the lifestyle habits above, rather than relying on claims on a label.

15 Foods that Boost the Immune System

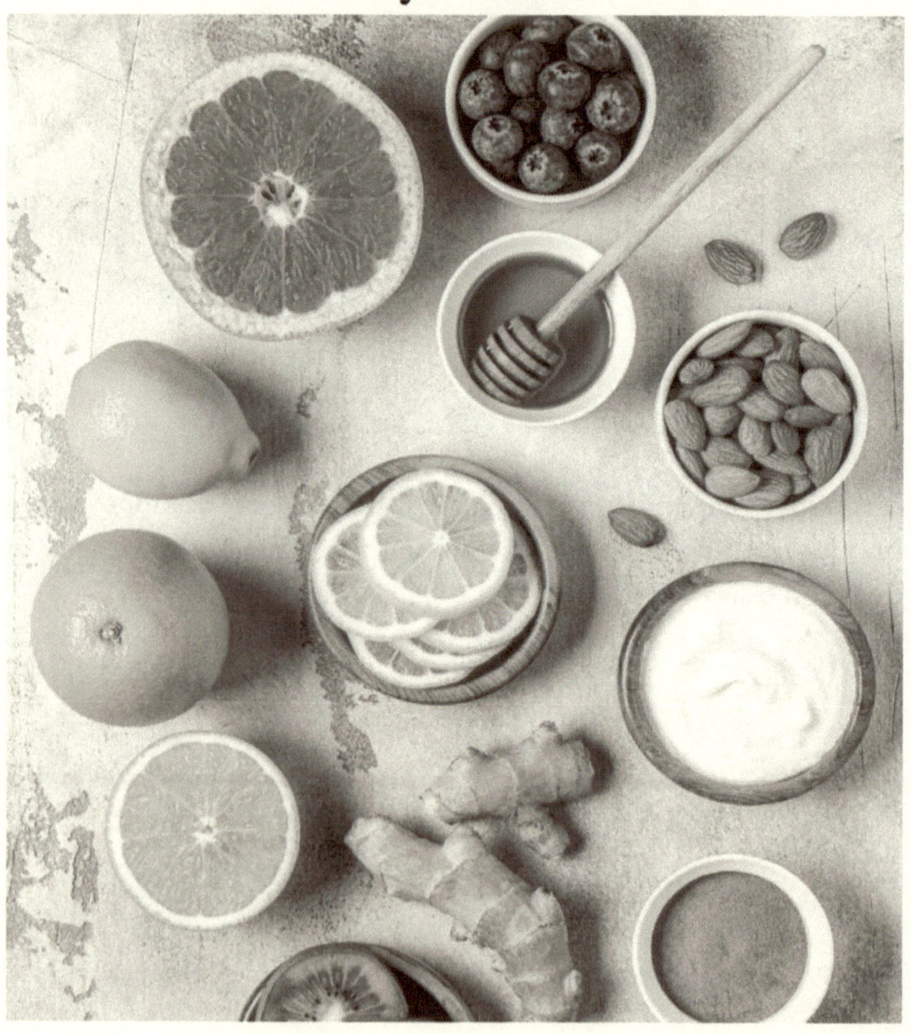

Immune system boosters

Feeding your body certain foods may help keep your immune system strong.

If you're looking for ways to prevent colds, the flu, and other infections, your first step should be a visit to your local grocery store. Plan your meals to include these 15 powerful immune system boosters.

1. Citrus fruits

Most people turn straight to vitamin C after they've caught a cold. That's because it helps build up your immune system.

Vitamin C is thought to increase the production of white blood cells, which are key to fighting infections.

Almost all citrus fruits are high in vitamin C. With such a variety to choose from, it's easy to add a squeeze of this vitamin to any meal.

Popular citrus fruits include:

grapefruit

oranges

clementines

tangerines

lemons

limes

Because your body doesn't produce or store it, you need daily vitamin C for continued health. The recommended daily amount for most adults is:

75 mg for women

90 mg for men

If you opt for supplements, avoid taking more than 2,000 milligrams (mg) a day.

Also keep in mind that while vitamin C might help you recover from a cold quicker, there's no evidence yet that it's effective against the new coronavirus, SARS-CoV-2.

2. Red bell peppers

If you think citrus fruits have the most vitamin C of any fruit or vegetable, think again. Ounce for ounce, red bell peppers contain almost 3 times as much vitamin C (127 mgTrusted Source) as a Florida orange (45 mgTrusted Source). They're also a rich source of beta carotene.

Besides boosting your immune system, vitamin C may help you maintain healthy skin. Beta carotene, which your body converts into vitamin A, helps keep your eyes and skin healthy.

3. Broccoli

Broccoli is supercharged with vitamins and minerals. Packed with vitamins A, C, and E, as well as fiber and many other antioxidants, broccoli is one of the healthiest vegetables you can put on your plate.

The key to keeping its power intact is to cook it as little as possible — or better yet, not at all. ResearchTrusted Source has shown that steaming is the best way to keep more nutrients in the food.

4. Garlic

Garlic is found in almost every cuisine in the world. It adds a little zing to food and it's a must-have for your health.

Early civilizations recognized its value in fighting infections. Garlic may also slow down hardening of the arteries, and there's weak evidence that it helps lower blood pressure.

Garlic's immune-boosting properties seem to come from a heavy concentration of sulfur-containing compounds, such as allicin.

5. Ginger

Ginger is another ingredient many turn to after getting sick. Ginger may help decrease inflammation, which can help reduce a sore throat and inflammatory illnesses. Ginger may help with nausea as well.

While it's used in many sweet desserts, ginger packs some heat in the form of gingerol, a relative of capsaicin.

Ginger may also decrease chronic painTrusted Source and might even possess cholesterol-lowering propertiesTrusted Source.

6. Spinach

Spinach made our list not just because it's rich in vitamin C — it's also packed with numerous antioxidants and beta carotene, which may both increase the infection-fighting ability of our immune systems.

Similar to broccoli, spinach is healthiest when it's cooked as little as possible so that it retains its nutrients. However, light cooking makes it easier to absorb the vitamin A and allows other nutrients to be released from oxalic acid, an antinutrient.

7. Yogurt

Look for yogurts that have the phrase "live and active cultures" printed on the label, like Greek yogurt. These cultures may stimulate your immune system to help fight diseases.

Try to get plain yogurts rather than the kind that are flavored and loaded with sugar. You can sweeten plain yogurt yourself with healthy fruits and a drizzle of honey instead.

Yogurt can also be a great source of vitamin D, so try to select brands fortified with this vitamin. Vitamin D helps regulate the immune system and is thought to boost our body's natural defenses against diseases.

Clinical trials are even in the works to study its possible effects on COVID-19.

8. Almonds

When it comes to preventing and fighting off colds, vitamin E tends to take a backseat to vitamin C. However, this powerful antioxidant is key to a healthy immune system.

It's a fat-soluble vitamin, which means it requires the presence of fat to be absorbed properly. Nuts, such as almonds, are packed with the vitamin and also have healthy fats.

Adults only need about 15 mg of vitamin E each day. A half-cup serving of almonds, which is about 46 whole, shelled almonds, provides around 100 percentTrusted Source of the recommended daily amount.

9. Sunflower seeds

Sunflower seeds are full of nutrients, including phosphorous, magnesium, and vitamins B-6 and E.

Vitamin E is important in regulating and maintaining immune system function. Other foods with high amounts of vitamin E include avocados and dark leafy greens.

Sunflower seeds are also incredibly high in selenium. Just 1 ounce contains nearly halfTrusted Source the selenium that the average adult needs daily. A variety of studies, mostly performed on animals, have looked at its potential to combat viral infections such as swine flu (H1N1).

10. Turmeric

You may know turmeric as a key ingredient in many curries. This bright yellow, bitter spice has also been used for years as an anti-inflammatory in treating both osteoarthritis and rheumatoid arthritis.

ResearchTrusted Source shows that high concentrations of curcumin, which gives turmeric its distinctive color, can help decrease exercise-induced muscle damage. Curcumin has promise as an immune booster (based on findings from animal studies) and an antiviral. More research is needed.

11. Green tea

Both green and black teas are packed with flavonoids, a type of antioxidant. Where green tea really excels is in its levels of epigallocatechin gallate (EGCG), another powerful antioxidant.

In studies, EGCG has been shown to enhance immune function. The fermentation process black tea goes through destroys a lot of the EGCG. Green tea, on the other hand, is steamed and not fermented, so the EGCG is preserved.

Green tea is also a good source of the amino acid L-theanine. L-theanine may aid in the production of germ-fighting compounds in your T cells.

12. Papaya

Papaya is another fruit loaded with vitamin C. You can find doubleTrusted Source the daily recommended amount of vitamin C in a single medium fruit. Papayas also have a digestive enzyme called papain that has anti-inflammatory effects.

Papayas have decent amounts of potassium, magnesium, and folate, all of which are beneficial to your overall health.

13. Kiwi

Like papayas, kiwis are naturally full of a ton of essential nutrients, including folate, potassium, vitamin K, and vitamin C.

Vitamin C boosts the white blood cells to fight infection, while kiwi's other nutrients keep the rest of your body functioning properly.

14. Poultry

When you're sick and you reach for chicken soup, it's more than just the placebo effect that makes you feel better. The soup may help lower inflammation, which could improve symptoms of a cold.

Poultry, such as chicken and turkey, is high in vitamin B-6. About 3 ounces of light turkey or chicken meat contains nearly one-third of your daily recommended amount of B-6.

Vitamin B-6 is an important player in many of the chemical reactions that happen in the body. It's also vital to the formation of new and healthy red blood cells.

Stock or broth made by boiling chicken bones contains gelatin, chondroitin, and other nutrients helpful for gut healing and immunity.

15. Shellfish

Shellfish isn't what jumps to mind for many who are trying to boost their immune system, but some types of shellfish are packed with zinc.

Zinc doesn't get as much attention as many other vitamins and minerals, but our bodies need it so that our immune cells can function as intended.

Varieties of shellfish that are high in zinc include:

oysters

crab

lobster

mussels

Keep in mind that you don't want to have more than the daily recommended amount of zinc in your diet:

11 mg for adult men

8 mg for most adult women

Too much zinc can actually inhibit immune system function.

16. More ways to prevent infections

Variety is the key to proper nutrition. Eating just one of these foods won't be enough to help fight off the flu or other infections, even if you eat it constantly. Pay attention to serving sizes and recommended daily intake so that you don't get too much of a single vitamin and too little of others.

Eating right is a great start, and there are other things you can do to protect you and your family from the flu, cold, and other illnesses.

Workout During the Coronavirus Pandemic

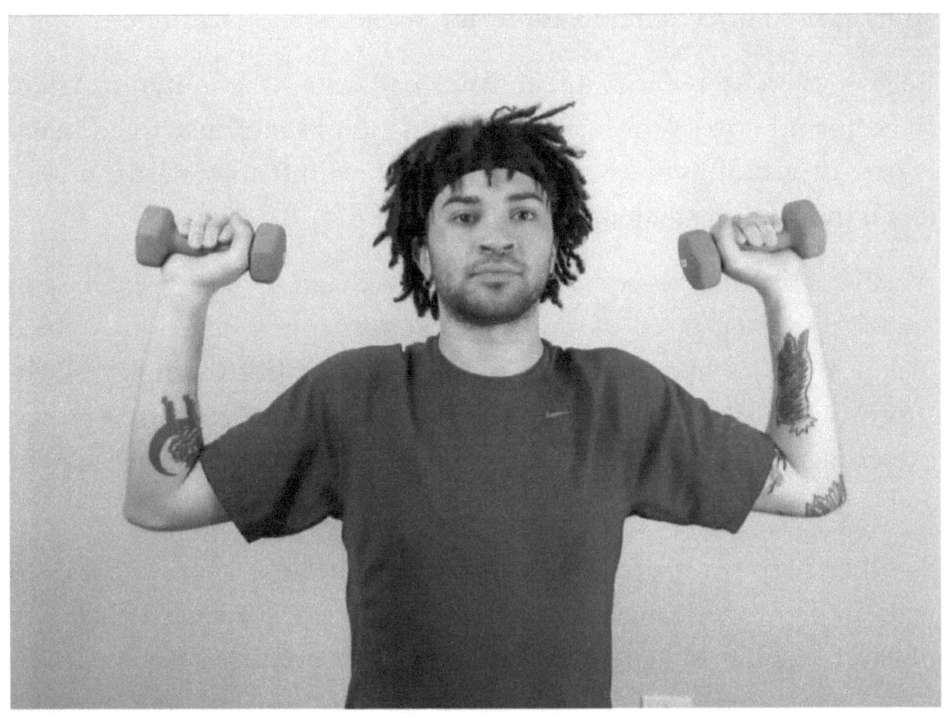

Exercise has many proven health benefits, from reducing the risk of cardiovascular disease to improving your mood — and even a stronger immune system.

There are many theories as to how exercise boosts the immune system, and it's likely that this happens in a few different ways. Here's what you need to know, and how you can exercise safely during the coronavirus pandemic.

Exercise boosts immunity and can help fight off infections

Exercise benefits your immune system in many ways. It can increase blood flow, help clear bacteria out of your airways, cause a brief elevation in body temperature that may be protective, strengthen antibodies to help fight infection, and reduce stress hormones.

Regular exercise reduces inflammation, allowing the immune system to perform better. While acute inflammation in response to an injury is part of a healthy immune system, chronic inflammation can slow down the immune system.

A 2019 scientific review found that moderate-intensity exercise is linked to lower rates of upper respiratory tract infections, which includes viruses like the flu and common cold. For example, a 2018 study of 1413 people in China found that those who reported exercising at least three times a week reduced their likelihood of getting a cold by 26%.

Another 2018 study of 390 people found that those who were trained with an eight-week regimen of moderate exercise reduced their risk of acute respiratory illness by 14%, and their number of sick days by 23%, compared with people who did not receive the exercise training.

How to exercise safely during the coronavirus pandemic

According to guidelines from the Centers for Disease Control and Prevention (CDC), healthy adults should aim to get at least 150 minutes of moderate exercise each week — which can include activities like walking, yoga, or gardening.

But even small amounts of exercise can help strengthen your immune system. "As little as an additional 10 minutes of walking a day or

1,000 steps can have a huge impact," Marvasti says.

Exercising during the pandemic can be tricky with stay-at-home orders in place and gyms closed. And Scott says it's most important that you follow social-distancing guidelines — exercise can help build your immunity and response, but it won't totally prevent you from getting sick if you are directly exposed to germs.

Scott also emphasizes that there are plenty of worthy exercises you can do inside and at home, including:

Chair exercises:

Similar to the last exercise, seated leg holds involve the same movement, but instead holding your legs in the same place, making them an isometric exercise.

Again, 30 seconds, one minute, or two minutes are the recommended levels.

Do this exercise three to five times a day for best results, either continuously or spaced throughout the day.

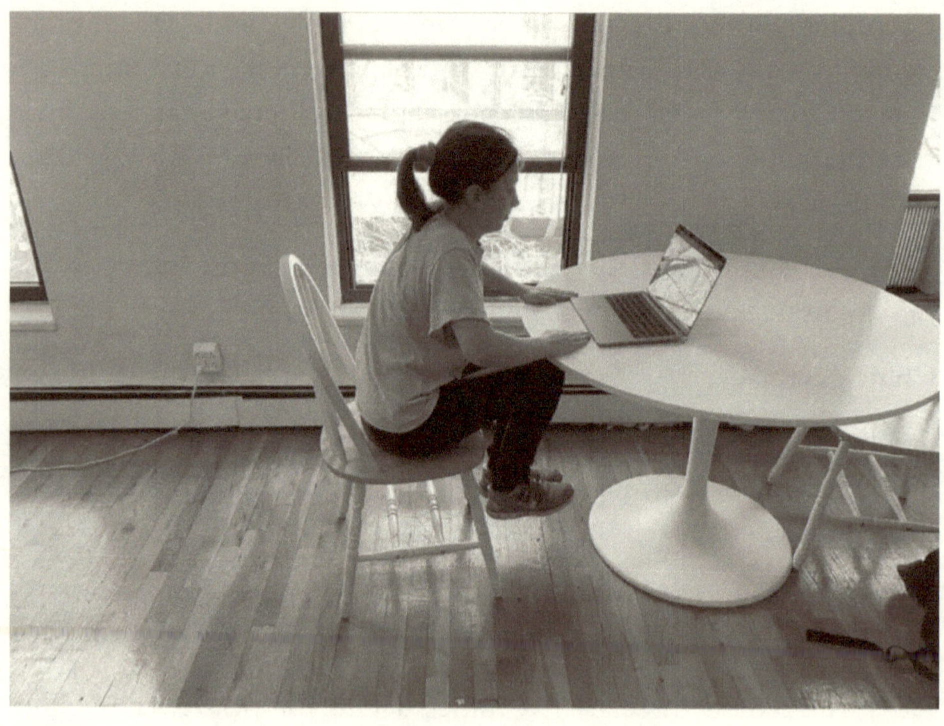

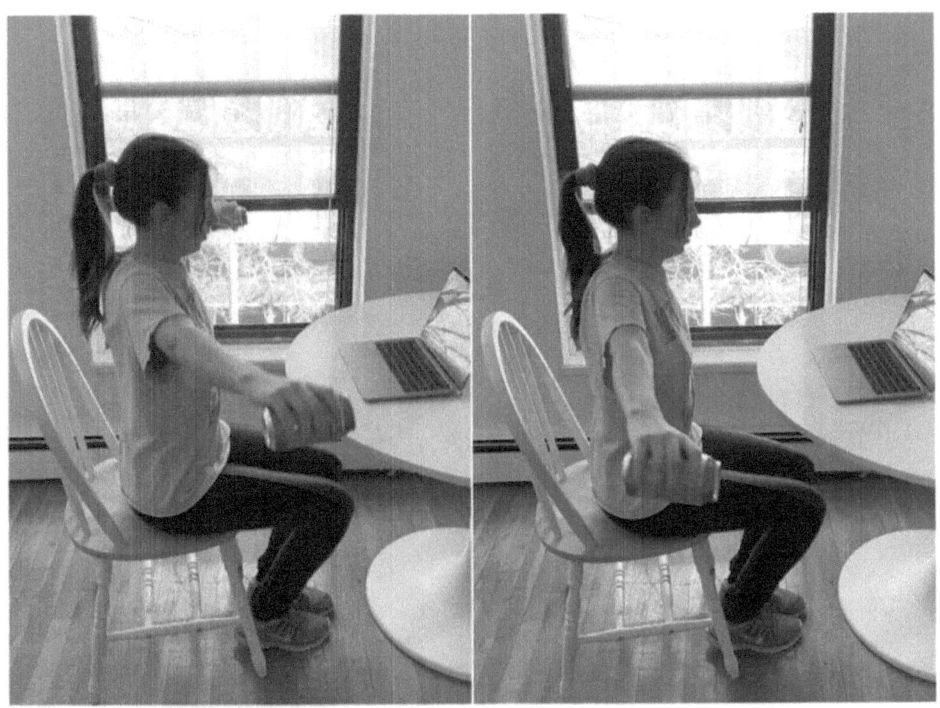

The seated shoulder exercise was simple to learn, and you can use anything you have on hand that weighs one to two pounds.

In each hand, grab pencils, bottles of water, or anything that has the equivalence of 1- to 2-pound dumbbells. Then lift your arms on each side, fully extended and parallel to the floor, with the back of your hands facing the ceiling. Now you are going to do little circles with your hands until it really burns, then you switch to small up and downs motion until you really can't hold it anymore. This is plyometric contraction

Try this for 30 seconds, one minute, or 90 seconds.

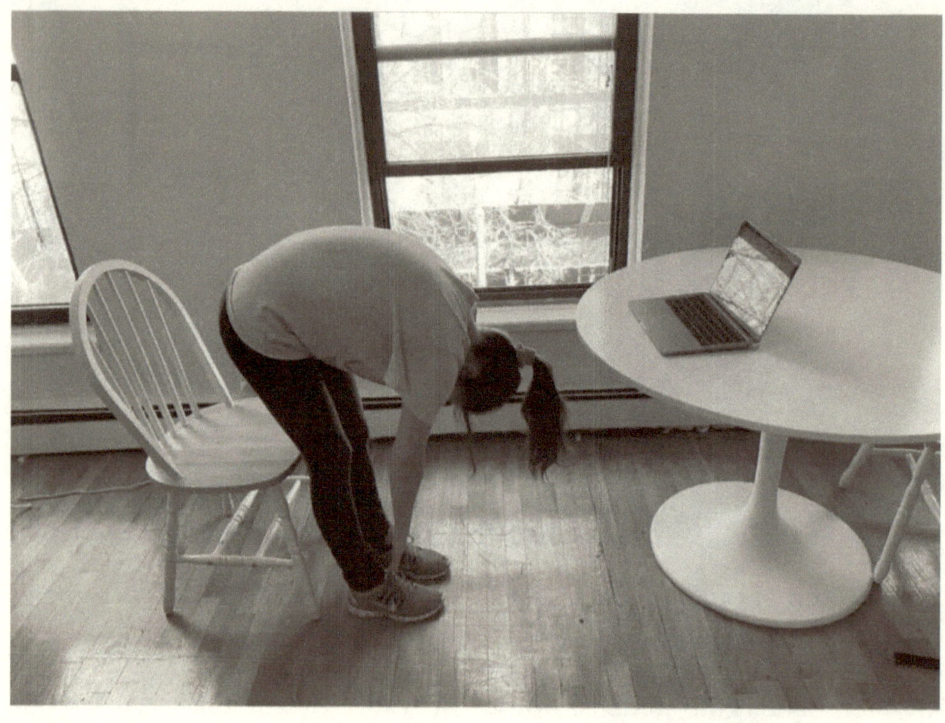

Stand up, then try to touch your toes while keeping your legs straight. If you can only reach your mid-calves, it's OK. Make sure that you are locking out your knees, keeping your legs straight, and feeling the stretch on the nerves behind the knees

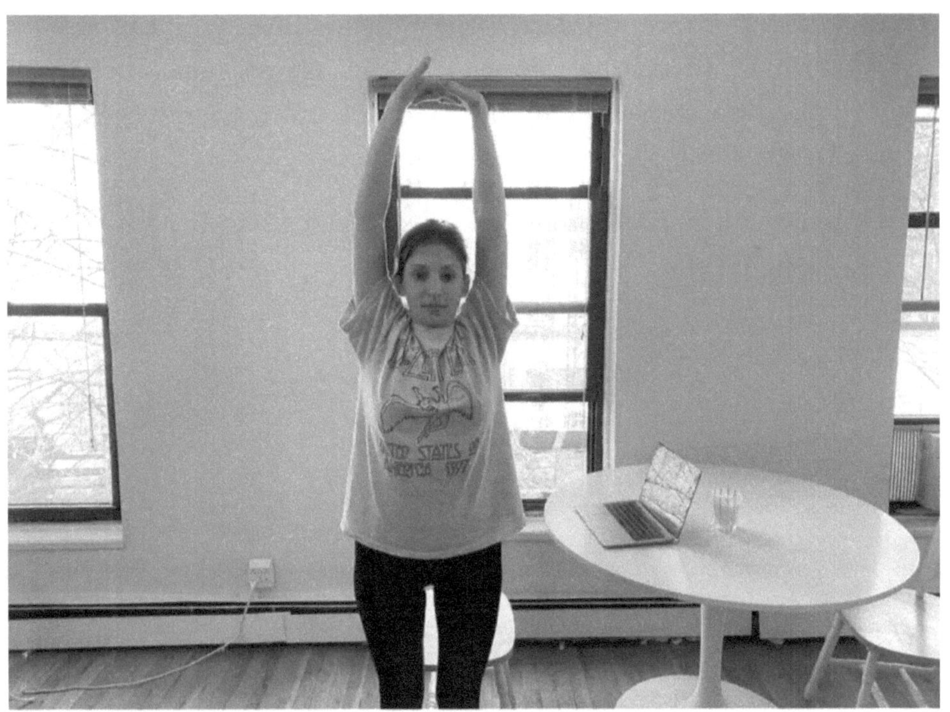

Cross your fingers, push your hands towards the ceiling to try to become as tall as possible, then do some torso rotation to the left, and to the right (10 rotations each side), keep your arms up and slowly push your left hip to the left, while your hands point to the right, to shift your pelvis on the side and stretch your oblique muscles, then do same thing on the right side

o be healthy, you need to get your heart rate at least once a week above 160 to 180 BPM, lift weights, work on your core, and stretch.

Resistance band exercises: If you are unable to go to the gym, resistance bands are a relatively inexpensive option to build strength and stability and improve heart health while working out at home.

Resistance bands are rubbery, elastic bands that you can use to strengthen your muscles at home. You can use resistance bands for many types of exercises that can help you tone your whole body using a relatively simple piece of equipment.

Here's what you need to know about resistance band workouts and how you can use them at home.

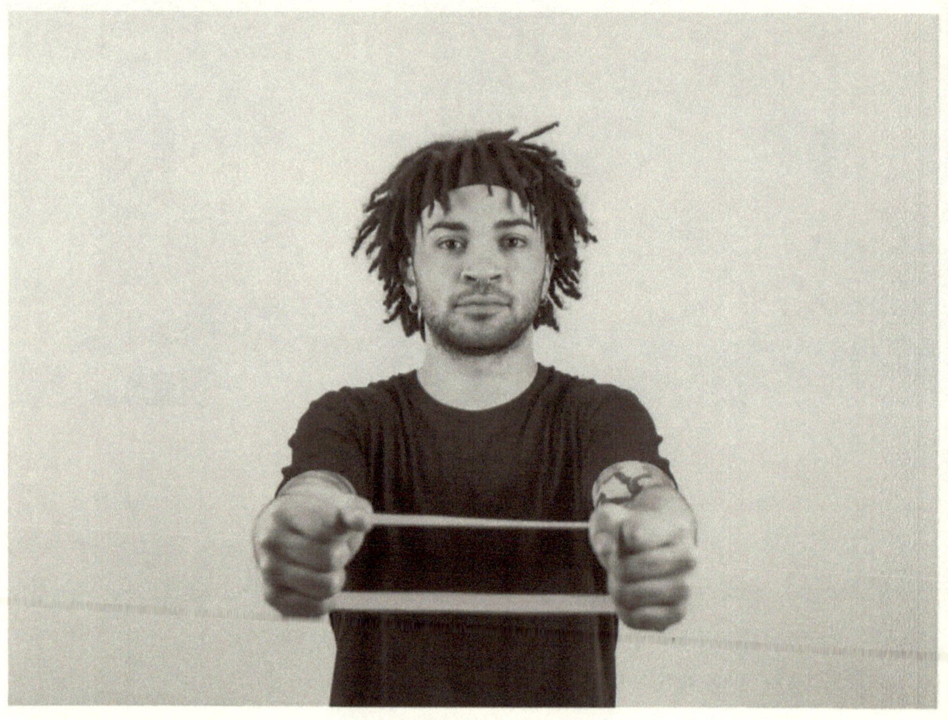

A workout guide

Resistance training is any type of exercise that uses resistance or weight to build strength in your muscles. Working out with resistance bands is one option for resistance training that allows you to work out at home using just one piece of equipment.

You can do many types of workouts using resistance bands, allowing you to tone muscles in your arms, legs, and core. Below are three resistance band workouts that you can try at home.

1. Alternating arm and leg: This exercise works out your core muscles including your abdominal and gluteal muscles.

Pull-on the resistance band so that it sits above both knees.

Get on your hands and knees in a tabletop position.

Reach one hand forward while kicking the opposite foot back.

Return to tabletop, then repeat on the other side.

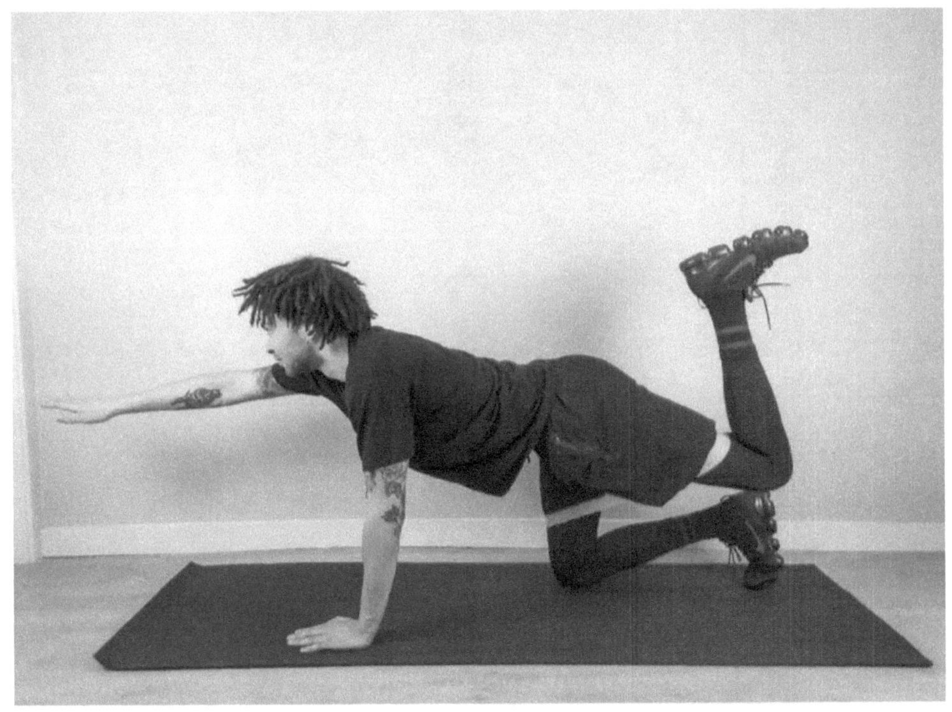

Alternating arm and leg tones the abs and glutes.

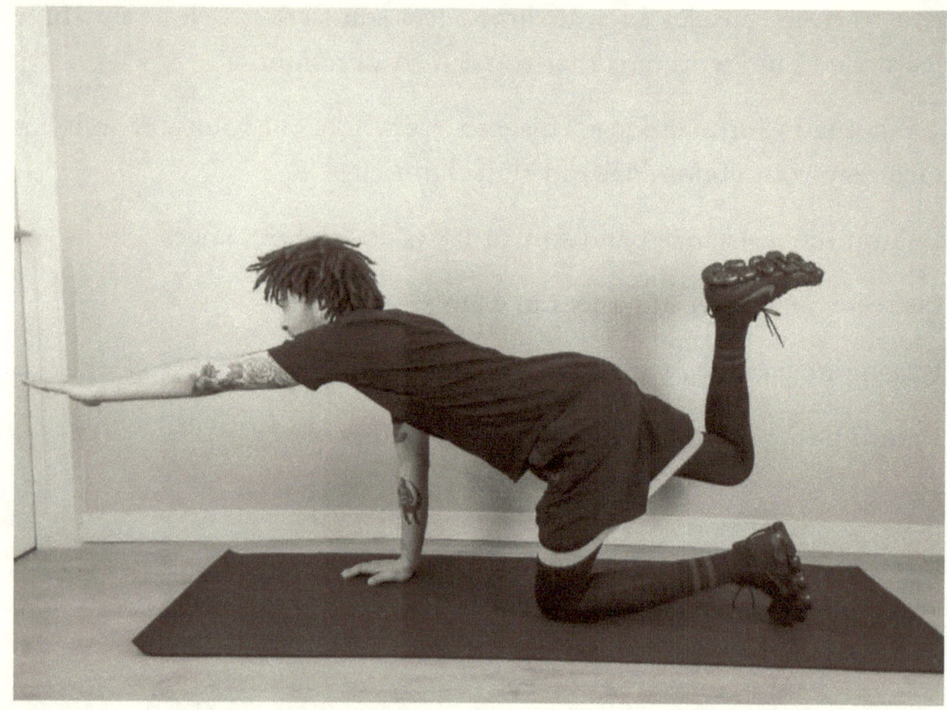

Maintain a tabletop position for proper form.

2. Bicep curl: This exercise targets your biceps and can be done either standing or sitting.

Wrap the band under your right foot if standing or under your right knee if you're sitting.

Hold the ends of the band out in front of you in your right hand, with your right elbow against your side and our fist facing upward.

Pull your hand upward toward your right shoulder while keeping your elbow in the same position.

Release your arm and bring it back down, then repeat on the left side.

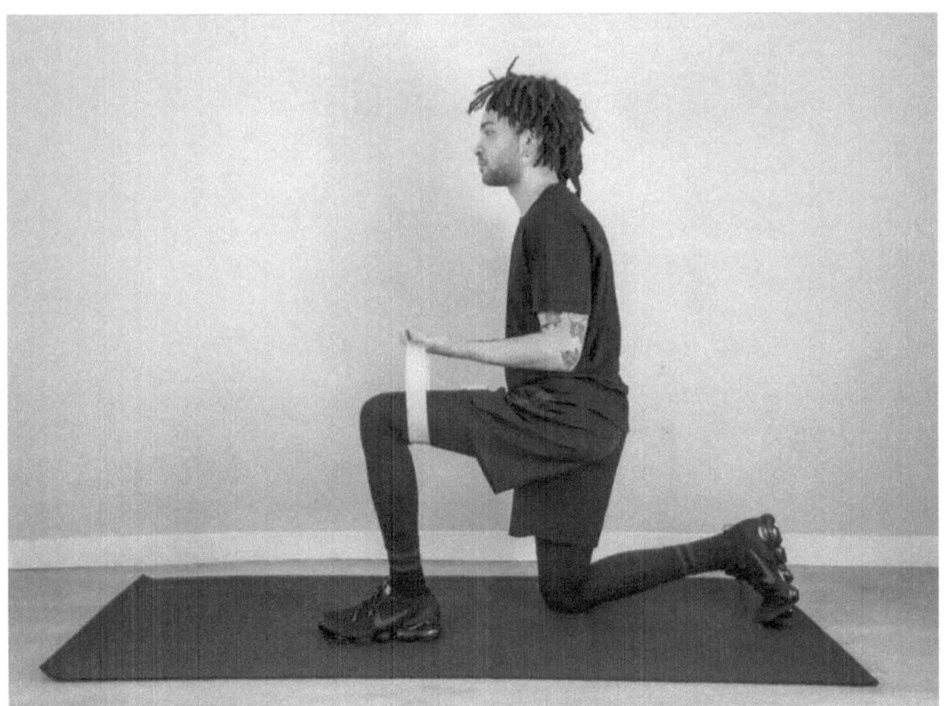

You don't need weights to tone your biceps.

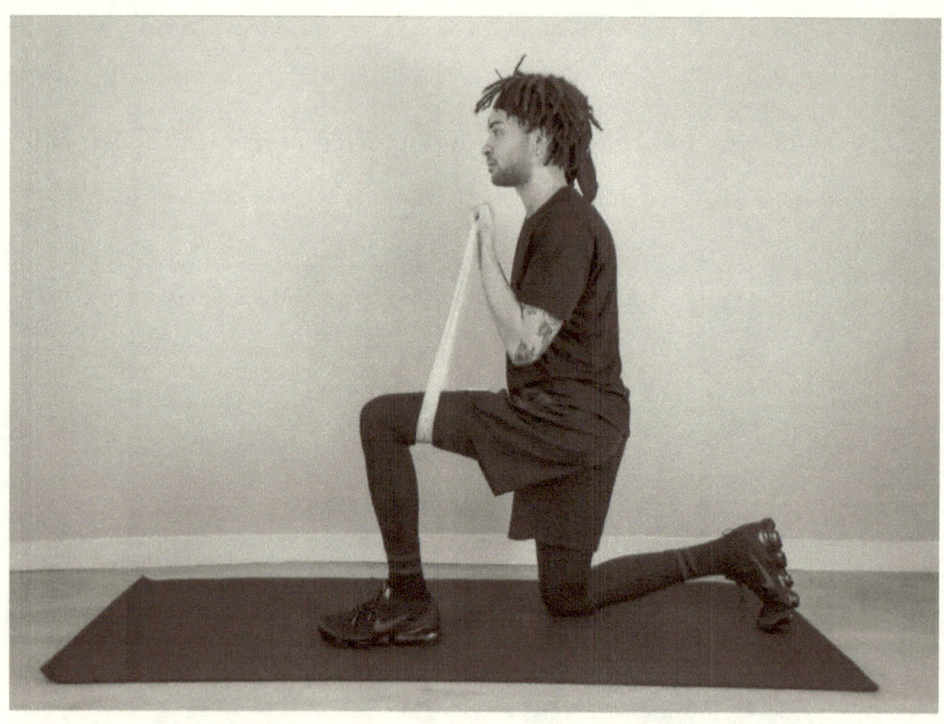

3. Squat: This tones your thighs and gluteal muscles.

Stand in a squat position with feet shoulder-width apart and the resistance band around your thighs.

Bend your knees into a squat while at the same time pulling your knees slightly apart to create tension.

Rise back up and repeat.

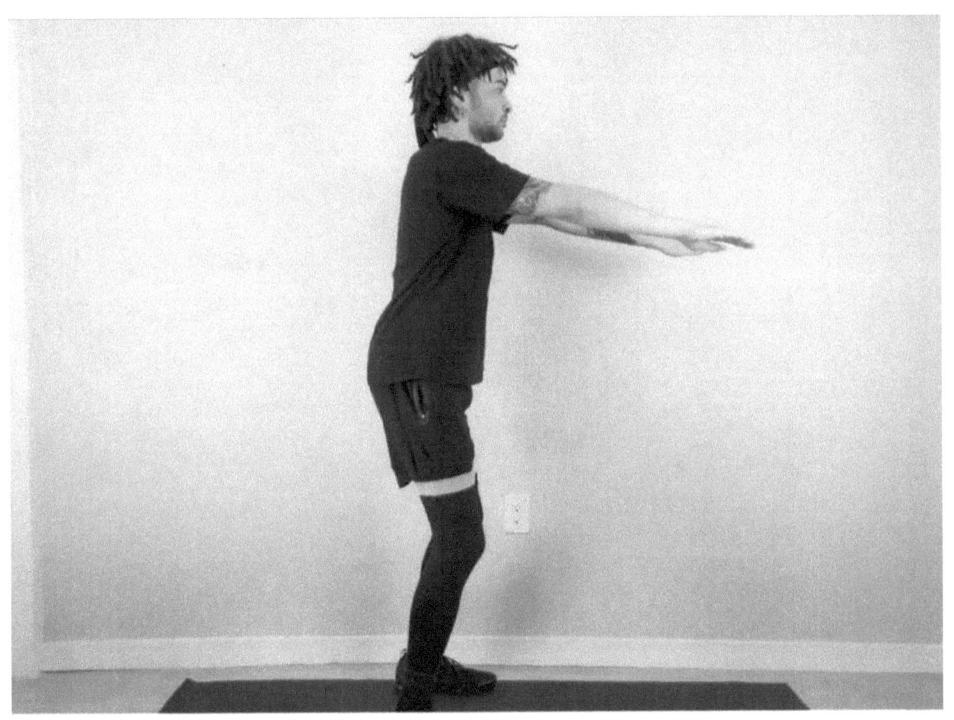

Squats with resistance bands are a great way to tone your thighs.

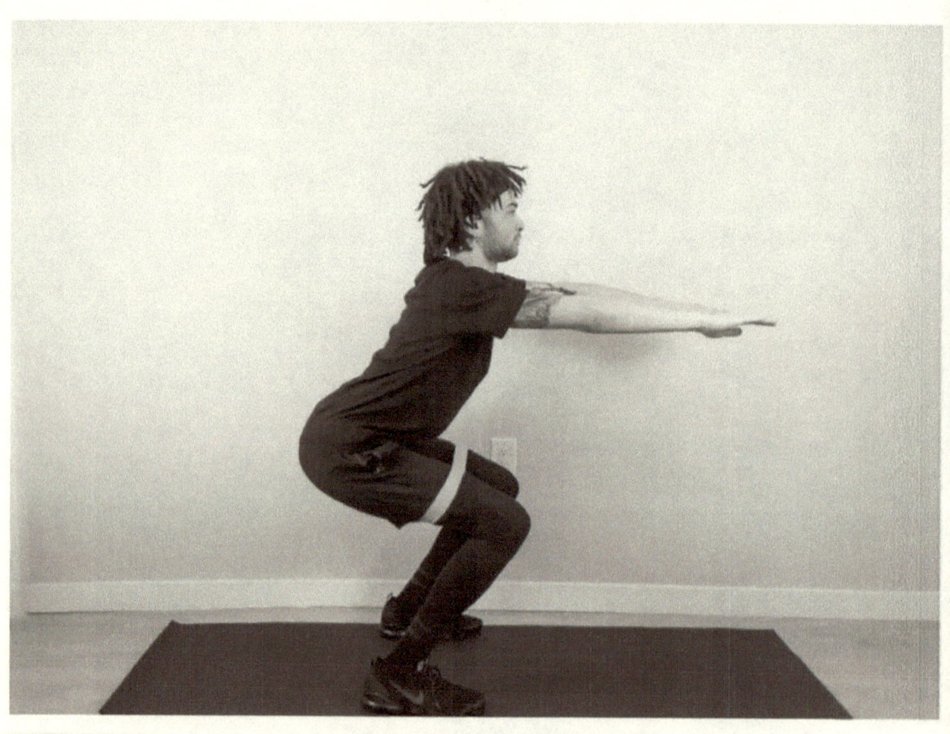

You should feel resistance against your thighs as you settle into the squat.

Isometric exercises

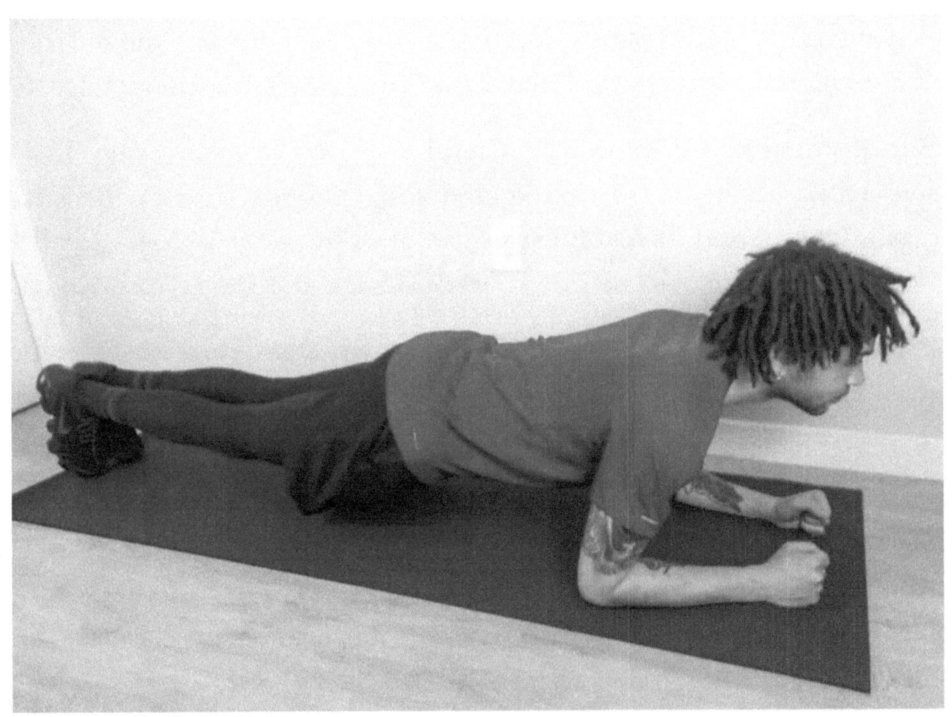

Isometrics are low-impact exercises that strengthen muscles through holding poses. Plank holds and many other poses common to yoga, barre, or pilates are examples of isometric exercises.

You'll know the exercise is isometric when it's done in one position where the specific muscle is tensed and held in that flexed position for at least six seconds. While they are low-impact and therefore put less strain on your body, there are limits to what isometrics can do.

Here's what you need to know about who can benefit from isometrics and some examples of isometrics you can do at home.

Isometrics can be used in physical therapy

Anyone can benefit from isometrics, can be done to tone the muscles in conjunction with traditional weight-lifting or resistance training.

But isometrics are especially useful for people recovering from surgery or an injury that's required long periods of rest. Because during that period of rest muscles can atrophy — or become smaller — which then need to be slowly worked back into shape, says Kolba.

Isometric exercises allow people to target areas that need to be strengthened without straining weak or injured joints, which makes them good for people who have suffered knee injuries, for example. Because the injured knee joint is restricted from movement but the muscle is still worked through the tension.

Isometrics are also good exercise for people suffering from rheumatoid arthritis and can be used to help treat people with hypertension.

Isometric exercises you can do at home

Isometrics are a great workout you can do at home because the only equipment you need is your own body weight and, sometimes, a stable wall. Here are some examples of popular isometric exercises.

Plank Hold: Planking works your midsection, shoulders and quad muscles of your legs. It should not be performed by people with shoulder or neck injuries.

Lay down on a yoga mat on your belly and then lift yourself up horizontally onto your toes and forearms.

Flex your abs, core, and glutes and hold that flex for 6 to 15 seconds.

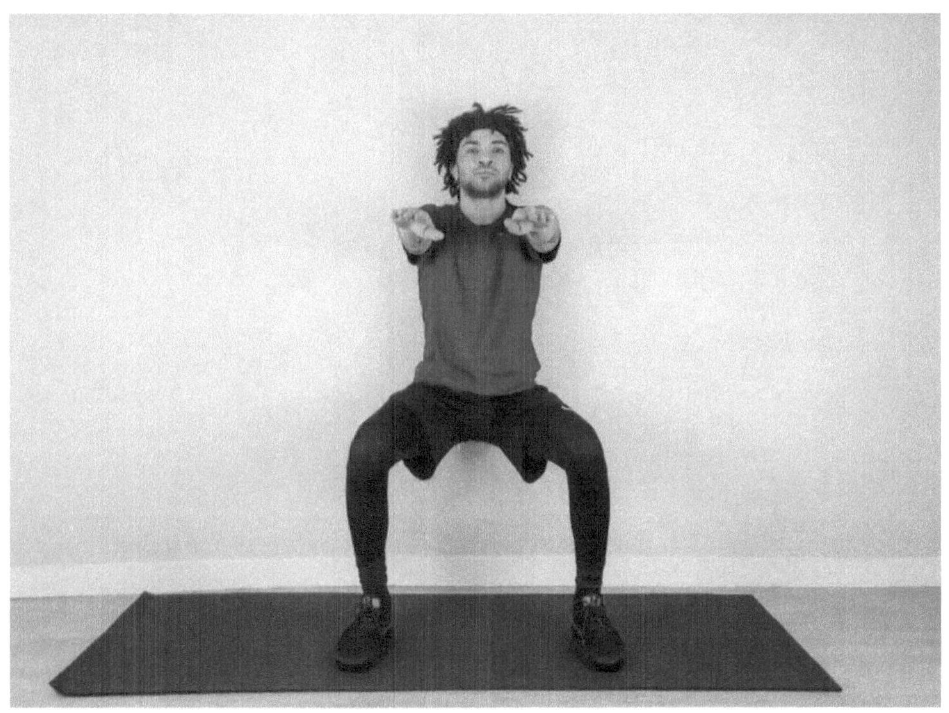

Wall Sit: This exercise strengthens the legs, especially the glutes, quadriceps, and hamstrings. This exercise will strengthen the hips as well and help with balance.

Stand about 2 feet, or so, from the wall.

Lean back so your back is flat against the wall and slide down slowly until your thighs are parallel to the ground in a sitting position while pressing against the wall.

While in this sitting position, flex your legs tightly and hold this position for 6 to 15 seconds.

Many states are allowing residents to get outside to exercise. Just remember, if you do exercise outside, be sure to leave at least six feet of space between you and anyone else.

In addition, having an accountability partner can help you exercise more often, and it's still possible to have a workout buddy these days.